Workout Philosophy

Workout Plans To Build Muscles, Break Mind Barriers And Eliminates Insecurities

Introduction

This book has actionable information on how to build muscles, break mind barriers and eliminate insecurities by following a new workout philosophy guaranteed to enable you to see results.

Motivation Is Good, But Drive Kills Motivation"
"Unknown:

Would you like to start working out but would like a new approach and methodology that is more efficient and effective? Or are you sick of the same old tired approach that doesn't seem to get the results you desire? Did you know that by simply adjusting your approach to working out, you could make a huge difference?

This book aims at giving you a new and better way of looking at the process of working out. For instance, you will understand why working out until you become tired and uncomfortable and then following up with a long period of rest is a lot better than the common approach of relying on a definite workout routine where you perform a specific number of repetitions.

I will also depict how motivation and drive, two closely related concepts, are actually different and how you can use that knowledge to improve your results while working out.

Additionally, we will look at specific workout techniques and how you can implement them in the new recommended style. Afterwards, I will show you how these techniques will not only help you gain muscle and stay fit, but also help fight stress and insecurity.

By the time you are done with this book, you will have figured out a new and smarter way of going about your workouts that will provide you with an edge against the vast majority of people who are doing the opposite.

Are you ready? Great, let's begin.

Thanks again for purchasing this book. I hope you enjoy it!

Table of Contents

Drive or Motivation and Their Place in Working Out

Let's begin our discussion by looking at how drive and motivation are different from each other.

If you are like most people, you probably make the erroneous assumption that drive and motivation mean the same thing. Well, apparently, that notion is wrong. And in this chapter, we will see why.

First, let us define the word "motivation". In simple terms, motivation can be described as the willingness you have for doing something. For instance, you could have a willingness to apply for a certain position. Also, you could have a willingness to travel to some place. At the same time, you could have a willingness to love someone.

Most of the time, motivation is fueled by desire. You could have a burning desire for someone. You could have a desire for touring different places around the world. You could desire to hold a certain position at work. That desire fuels the willingness to take the appropriate steps to accomplish the goal you have in mind.

Then we have what is known as "drive". So what is drive really?

In the context of accomplishing goals or performing certain actions, Merriam Webster defines drive as the state of being under pressure or feeling hurried.

If you think about it, drive can also make you accomplish goals. For instance, picture yourself working at a job that provides you with a deadline. Now imagine that the deadline is approaching and that you realize that you are barely halfway past the project you are working on.

How would you feel?

Imagine the amount of stress and anxiety that would build within you. It gets even worse if the consequences for not delivering would be grave, such as getting fired. This situation will put you under tremendous amount of pressure and you will find yourself doing everything you can to finish your project.

That is the impact drive can have on you.

What point am I trying to make here? Well, all that I am saying is that motivation and drive can both compel you to take action. But the reasons behind your actions are utterly different.

Motivation compels you to take action based on positive energy and desire - your desire for becoming a better person, your desire for earning more money, your desire for recognition.

Drive, on the other hand, pushes you to take action from a position of fear, stress and apprehension – your fear of job loss, your fear of not having enough money, your fear of losing your health, your fear of being alone, or your fear of failure.

Is this difference starting to make sense to you?

Let us now look at how this difference applies to your workout endeavors.

Motivation and Drive As It Applies To Working Out

In many ways, motivation and drive apply to most areas of your life. And that includes working out.

Let me ask you a question; are you motivated to work out or are you driven?

If you have been keen on my explanation in the previous chapter, hopefully, you get the idea. If, for some reason you still don't, this chapter will help you straighten things out.

Believe it or not, the reasons behind you working out or choosing to start working out could not be what you think. You will need to spend some time on self-reflection to understand the force behind your actions.

Maybe your workplace has implemented a workout routine for its employees as a means to help you achieve better health. In this case, you are not working out because you want to; you are do so only because you are being forced to. It is a must.

The same goes for when you are working out as a means of trying to fit in. If all of your closest friends are regularly working out and are in their best of shapes as a result, you may feel compelled to start doing the same for fear of being the odd one out. So, you put yourself under a lot of pressure to work out, not because of your own willingness to do so, but because of wanting to belong.

The situation is quite different when you want to work out purely because you are motivated to do so. Maybe after purchasing the latest issue of Men's Health magazine, you felt inspired. You desired the beach bodies you saw on the pictures. Then you vowed to yourself to do everything you could to get that kind of body.

In this case, you will have little difficulty approaching your workout. You will work out because you understand that it is in your best interest that you do so and the amount of stress you will experience will be considerable lower.

So, the bottom-line is, stressful events are the trigger of a drive.

Which Is Better? Is It Working Out Based Motivation Or Drive?

Now that you are able to tell the difference between motivation and drive and how it applies to working out, it is time that you moved past the basics and asked yourself the next important question, "Which way is better? Is it depending on your motivation or your drive?" Let us spend some time answering this question.

Interestingly, most of the workout routines out there are designed to drive you and not to motivate you. For instance, think about a workout session that requires that you to perform up to 20 pushups.

For some of us, this may not be a problem. You may be able to perform 20 pushups without breaking a sweat. Still, similarly, performing the same number of pushups may be difficult at best for others. If you think about it, there is a fundamental flaw in this type of workout routine. For one thing, if you are the kind of person who performs 20 pushups without battering an eyelid, then it means that this kind of task is an all too easy challenge for you.

Therefore, what this means that if you only perform this one routine as stated, you will barely get much value from it.

How do I know this? This is because according to Verywellfit, for a workout to be effective on the muscles, you need to work them until you get tired.

In other words, for your workout to be considered to be of good quality, you need to exert the maximum effort you possibly can on the muscles you are working. This is very unlikely if you are the kind of person who can do 20 push-ups with much ease. For your workout to be effective, you will probably need to do 20 more pushups.

On the other hand, if you find it difficult to perform the same number of push-ups, you will only be forcing your body to perform the workout mainly from a position of high pressure and stress, not because you desire to.

So, how do you go about it? Which way will best serve your interest?

Well, here is the verdict. The key to working out effectively is to work out until you feel your muscles have had enough but no further. Put differently, this means you work your muscles until they tire. After that, you can quit and have some rest.

So, thinking back to the example of the push-ups, if you are a strong person, this means that you could do more, perhaps forty even fifty before you experience exhaustion. Conversely, if you are weaker, you could perform ten or perhaps fifteen push-ups before choosing to rest.

The important thing is; you have to work out until you arrive the point of discomfort, then you quit. That point will vary from person to person but the important thing is that you reach that point. Counting numbers is not the slightest bit important in this case.

What Evidence Is There In Support Of It?

Obviously, this point of view is new to most of us. We are used to being told that we need to perform X number of sit-ups or X number of weight-lifts.

Therefore, if a new point of view surfaces suggesting otherwise, we are bound to question it.

However, I am not making this claim or recommendation lightly.

As it turns out, an interesting study carried out by researchers at the <u>Univeristy of Memphis</u>, has is in support of this new point of view. In the research, 38 subjects were classified under four categories.

One was made to perform 3-5 reps (keep in mind reps is shorthand for repetition), the second 13-15 reps, the third, 23-25 reps and a fourth that acted as a control to the experiment was subjected to no physical training. The study was conducted over a period of 7 weeks

As shocking as it may seem, the results depicted that the group that carried out 3-5 reps outperformed the rest.

So what is the point?

A lower rep is better than higher rep if you are looking to build muscle and get stronger, provided you focus to the point where your workout gets uncomfortable.

What this means is that, more often than not, one rep is way better than ten reps, provided you are well focused.

Also, counting the number of times you work out is of least importance provided your get to the point where your muscles become exhausted. Afterwards, you can follow with periods of rest and repeat the process.

Up until this point, we have covered the difference between working out based on your motivation as well as your drive. We have also seen how stressful situations create drive. In addition, we have seen that working out to the point where you get exhausted is much more important than counting the number of reps.

Next up, we are going to look at various compound workout techniques that you can start implementing right away. Get ready; this plane is about to take off.

Effective Compound Workout Techniques

This book would be useless if I went on and on talking about how working out in a certain way was better without taking the time to show you how to actually do it. For that reason, I will cover different compound workout techniques in this chapter to guide you by the hand and tell you what to do.

By compound, I mean that the workout exercises covered in this chapter will move several joints and work several different muscles at the same time. They are different from isolation exercises that focus on working only a single group of muscles at a time. Therefore, by performing these compound workout exercises, you'll be making the most of your time and effort.

So let's begin.

Exercise 1: The Squat

First, we will begin our discussion by looking at a common compound workout – the squat. It is quite simple but very effective, which makes for a very good starting point. This workout will work quite a number of muscles in your body namely: the muscles of the hips, thighs, buttocks, quadriceps femoris and hamstrings. It is especially useful in increasing the size of your legs and as a result increasing core strength.

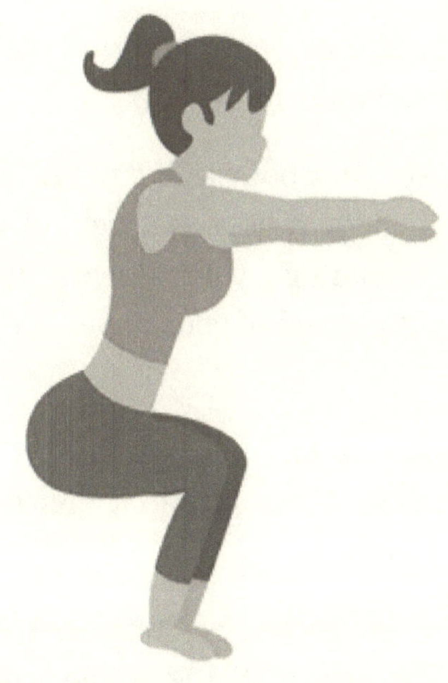

If you are interested in giving it a try, just follow the steps below:

1. Firstly, stand straight with your head facing directly ahead. As you do this, be sure to hold your chest up and let it protrude forward.

2. Then spread your legs out. Just let them be a hip-width apart as shown in the picture above.

3. Next, hold your hands stretched directly in front of you. This is meant to help you achieve balance as you carry out this exercise.

4. While in this position, begin making the muscles of your stomach tight. The way to do this is by pulling

back your shoulders, raising your chest and pulling the muscles of your abdomen in.

5. Now it is time to lower your body as if sitting. To do this right, imagine that there is a seat behind you. Start by slightly bending your knees while maintaining a straight posture of your upper body as much as possible.

    Also, as you do this, make sure that you knees don't move forward too much. Make sure that they don't move forward past your toes.

6. Now lift yourself in an attempt to straighten your legs. The key here is to ensure that your knees don't lock as you do this. Try to keep them apart as much as possible.

7. Lastly, repeat the steps above for as long as possible. Remember, the important thing is that you work out until you feel tired and uncomfortable; the number of times you repeat this exercise shouldn't be the focus. The important thing is that you accomplish the goal of feeling uncomfortable. Therefore, strive to push yourself to your own limits as much as you can.

Now you have learnt how to perform your first compound workout. As you've seen, it is nothing difficult as long as you have the willingness to do it.

Brace yourself because what follows are more techniques like this.

Exercise 2: Pushup To Overhead Press

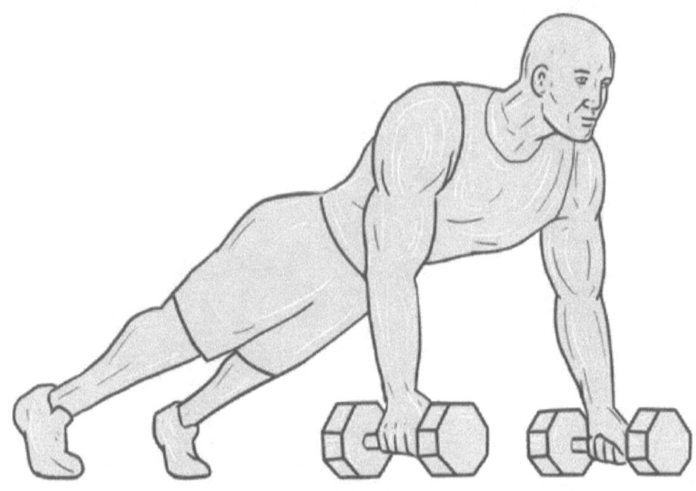

This compound workout technique is a combination of pushups and overhead dumbbell press. It is a fairly simple and effective exercise. It is especially good because it is known to target nearly every muscle group.

One of the best things about it is that you can use it whenever you find it difficult to keep up with your best workout routines either because you've been travelling, on holiday, working for so long, or whatever reasons you may be having. It is also good for you especially if you are not a big fan of strength training or you simply don't have enough space or equipment.

Because of these unique advantages, I like to regard it as a lifestyle hack. If you are interested in putting it into practice, below are the steps you need to follow:

1. Start by securing two dumbbells that you can lift overhead with good form. If you are a beginner to working out, this means that you should select dumbbells that fall in the 10 to 30 pounds weight range.

2. Get yourself in the ready position by standing with your feet about a shoulder-width apart and with the dumbbells close to your feet on the floor.

3. Now bend to a squat position, so that you can grab the dumbbells by your hands. To assume this position, you can follow the guidelines from the squat exercise we just covered. This means ensuring that you don't arch your back and maintaining your head in an upright position.

4. After holding the dumbbells by your hands, assume a pushup position as shown in the picture above. Then, perform one complete pushup.

5. Next, get back to the starting position with the dumbbells still in your hands. Use the squat position to lift your body to a standing position while holding the dumbbells at shoulder level.

6. Now it is time to perform the overhead press. With the dumbbells still held at should level, lift them above your head while stretching your arms such that your elbows are directly below the dumbbells as

show in the picture below. Afterwards, return the dumbbells to the starting position.

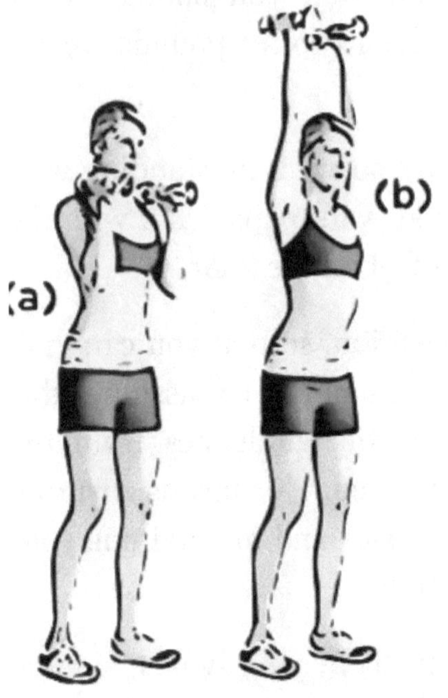

7. Now, lower the dumbbells to the level of your hips and then slowly squat. Remember to keep your head up and back straightened out. Place the dumbbells on the floor close to your feet.

8. The steps up to this point represent one rep of the pushup to overhead exercise. Your job at this point is to repeat steps 1 to 7 for as long as you possibly can. Once again, remember to quit when you become uncomfortable.

You have looked at yet another fairly effective compound exercise. There's more to discover along the way; just read on.

Exercise 3: Lunge

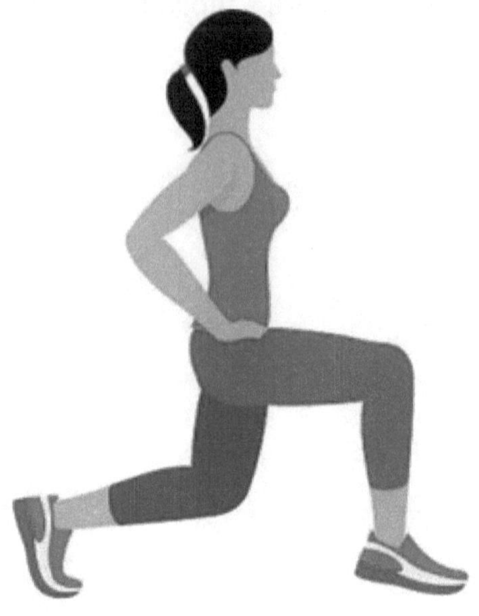

The Lunge is another compound workout technique that should be worth your attention. It is a surprisingly simple workout technique, which is especially good if you want to work the glutes in your thighs and butt. It is also useful for working the hamstring and quadriceps in the thighs.

The great thing about it is that you can perform it literally anywhere. Whether you are on a plane, at a beach, in your bedroom, at work or anywhere else and feel like working out, you'll have no qualms executing this technique.

1. First, begin at a standing position with your feet spread out a hip-width apart and place your hands on your waist.

2. In order to keep the upper part of your body straight, choose a spot or an object to stare at in front of you. Maintain your focus on it so that you do not look down.

3. Next, take a huge step forward.

4. While maintaining the majority of your weight on the front foot, slowly lower your hips.

5. Keep descending to the point where your back knee nearly touches the floor. At the same time, ensure that your front knee is directly above your ankle. Ideally, this should mean that both knees should form a $90°$ angle, as shown in the picture above.

6. Then press your front foot on the ground and slowly lift yourself back up to the starting position.

7. Lastly, switch your legs and perform steps 1 to six all over again. From now onwards, it's all a matter of switching legs and performing the same number of steps until you tire. Once you get to the point where it all gets uncomfortable, you can get some rest.

Performing lunges is arguably one of the best ways to challenge and work the muscles belonging to the lower body. However, you may quickly find out that this exercise strains your knees so much. If for some reason you end up feeling pain on your knees, you can reduce the size of your steps and slowly work your way increasing the size of your step as you get better.

With all that said, here are some things you should keep in mind as you perform this exercise:

- Avoid extending your knees beyond the level of the toes of the front foot.

- Don't let the knee on the rear foot touch the ground. Just let it hoover close to the ground while maintaining a 90° angle.

- Stop whenever you notice any pain on our knees before or during your performance.

- Keep your body straight and avoid leaning forward or backwards.

Are you eager to learn more? Keep reading to discover yet another amazing workout technique.

Exercise 4: Pull-Ups

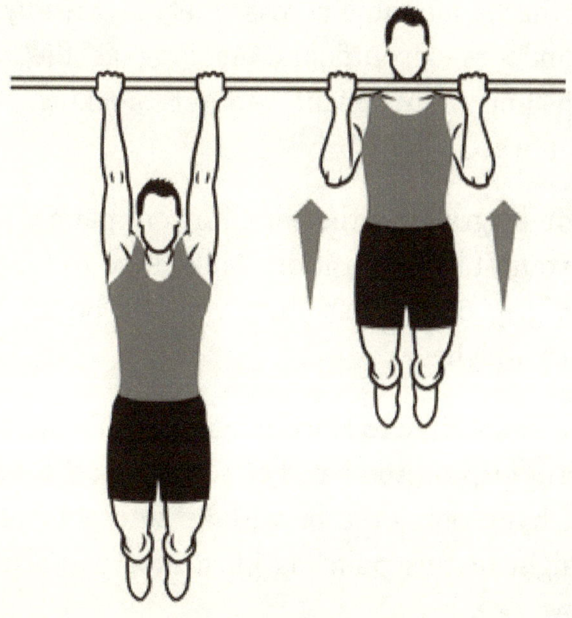

Now we get to talk about pull-ups. Unlike most workout techniques you've never heard of, pull-ups are quite commonplace. What may be news to you is the effectiveness of this exercise. Well, the fact of the matter is that pull-ups work muscles of the arms, shoulders, the scapular, abdomen and the pelvic floor. That is quite a large number of muscles worked by a single technique.

If you are interested in performing this exercise, it's actually quite simple. You just need to carry out the steps below:

1. First, you will need a pull-up bar. This can be any bar that is mounted across safely and firmly. It can be indoors or outdoors. As long as the bar can withstand your weight without breaking, you are good to go.

2. Begin by grabbing the bar with your palms. This will be your starting position. Make sure to maintain a firm grip on the bar since you will be lifting your entire weight.

3. Now is the time to start hanging. While maintaining a firm grip on the bar, get your feet off the ground and hang on to the bar. Make sure your arms are straight at this point as illustrated in the drawing above.

4. Next, start pulling yourself up. To do this, pull your elbows downwards as if bringing them to the ground. Consequently, with enough effort, you should be able to lift your body upwards.

5. Now, let yourself move all the way up to the point where your chin crosses the bar.

6. Next, slowly lower your body to the point where it is hanging, but with your arms straight.

7. The steps to this point represent one round. Now, your task will be to repeat the above steps until you get tired and uncomfortable. Then follow up with periods of rest.

As you can see, the steps for performing pull-ups are pretty simple and straightforward. Given enough time, pull-ups can start showing amazing results.

But wait, there's more. Would you like to achieve an amazing chest appearance? Up next, we talk about yet another compound exercise – the chest press.

Exercise 5: Chest Press

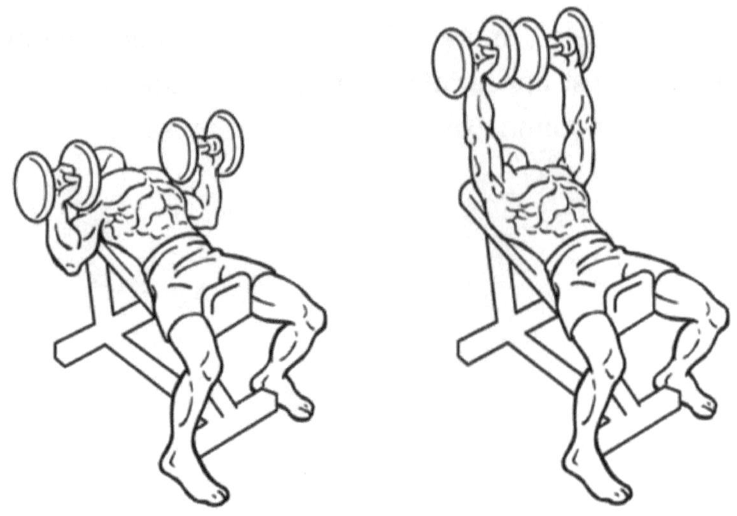

The chest press is particularly good for you if you intent on working your chest muscles. It is also good for working the muscles of the shoulder and the triceps. In this part, we will be looking at how you can implement this technique.

Normally, there are various ways of performing the chest press. However, for the purposes of this book, we will be looking at how you can carry out this technique using dumbbells. Therefore, the name of this technique is more accurately put as the dumbbell chest press.

The fact that we will be using dumbbells means that you are better off performing this exercise at the gym.

However, if you have gym equipment at home, then you can get started right away. That said, here are the steps you need to take.

1. First, lie on a bench and hold dumbbells with a strong grip at the center with both of your hands. Also, ensure that you plant your feet firmly in the ground.

2. Bring the dumbbells close to your chest and let them face each other, as shown in the illustration above. This position will represent your starting point.

3. Now take a huge and deep breath and press the dumbbells upwards to the point where they are directly above your chest and your arms are almost straight. Make sure that your hands are twisted such that your thumbs are placed side by side.

4. Take another deep breath and slowly bring the dumbbells down close to your chest, back to the starting position. You can do this on a count of 2.

5. At this point, you have completed one round of this technique. Now it is time to repeat steps 2 to 4 for as long as possible. As always, quit whenever you get tired and uncomfortable and get some quality rest.

As simple as this exercise sounds, there are a few points you should keep in mind if you are keen on doing it well and minimizing risk of injury. Keep the following in mind:

- Make sure you allow your back to keep a natural arch. This means that you should not let it lie completely flat on the bench. Allow a small gap to exist between your lower back and the bench.

- Avoid adjusting your body as you try to lift the weight. If you cannot avoid doing this, this is often a sign that you are lifting more weight than you can comfortably handle for this exercise. Ensure that you only lift weight that allows you to keep good form.

- As you press the dumbbells in an effort to lift them up, do so in a motion that resembles a triangle. It is not a requirement that the dumbbells touch each other.

There you have it. Now you know how to comfortably carry out the dumbbell chest press. Now let's talk about one last workout technique that you ought to know of – the crunch.

Exercise 6: The Crunch

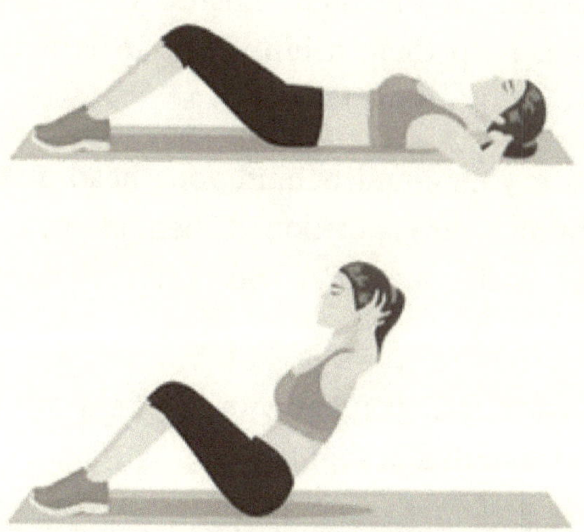

As we wind up our discussion of compound workout techniques, we will talk about a technique known as the crunch.

You no doubt have seen people with six pack abs. Have you ever admired them and wished that you could be like them? If so, you are in great luck. This technique is precisely what you will need to accomplish that goal.

Beyond merely working your abs, the crunch can also work your core and your spine. This helps you achieve good posture, balance and athletic performance.

And guess what; performing it isn't any complicated at all. You merely have to go through the steps that I will outline below.

Are you ready? Here are the steps:

1. First, lie flat on the floor. Ensure your knees are bent, then keep them a hip-width apart and plant your feet firmly on the floor.

2. Now place your hand behind your head such that your thumbs are positioned behind your ears. However, make sure that you don't interlace your fingers.

3. Next, ensure that your elbows are held out to the sides and rounded in slightly.

4. Tilt your chin towards your chest leaving out only a few inches of space.

5. Then pull the muscles of your abdomen inwards gently.

6. Now move forward as if sitting up so that your head, shoulders and neck are lifted off the floor.

7. Hold your position at the top of the movement and the slowly allow your body to move back to the floor.

8. Lastly, repeat the last two steps for as long as you are comfortable. When you get tired, quit and get some rest.

Good, now you know how to perform the crunch. There are a few things you need to keep in mind so that you do not end up injuring yourself or reducing the effectiveness of the exercise. They are:

- Avoid pulling your neck or drawing in your elbows. This will strain your neck and keep you from working your abs. Keep in mind that movement should come from your abs not your head.

- Don't crunch too high. Remember, the goal is not to sit up completely but to merely assume a similar position. Ideally, your shoulder blades should be lifted only a few inches from the floor.

- Relax as you bring yourself down to the floor. It is easier to allow your shoulders to fall off to the floor but that isn't what you should do. The goal should be to keep tension on the abs throughout the exercise. So do your best not to rest your shoulders on the floor completely.

Up to this point, we have covered the different compound workouts that you can put to use right away. We have also defined a new and better approach that involves working out until you get uncomfortable and tired instead of counting an exact number of reps.

I know you may still be wondering; how does this help you keep fit and relieve stress and insecurity? The next part of his book looks at that.

Why These Techniques Help With Stress And Insecurities

If you are struggling with stress and insecurity and are wondering how working out can help with that, you are in great company. According to the <u>Anxiety and Depression Association of America,</u> 7 out of 10 adults in the US reported experiencing stress and anxiety in their lives to the point where it affects their lives at least moderately. And this is according to a study done in 2008. My presumption is that as of now, the numbers are far much worse.

And keep in mind that insecurity mostly stems from a form of anxiety disorder known as <u>generalized anxiety disorder</u>. Therefore, insecurity is factored in within the numbers we have just discussed. This is to make you understand before anything else, that you are not alone.

This chapter will focus on showing you how working out helps alleviate the problems you currently have. First, we will begin by examining how working out helps fight stress. Afterwards, we will look at how it helps fight insecurity.

Without further ado, let's begin.

1. *How working out helps with stress*

The medical fraternity is convinced beyond reasonable doubt that any form of exercise can be used as a remedy against stress.

To begin, <u>Harvard health</u> provides some insights into how this works scientifically. It is argued that much of it has to do with how exercise affects the chemicals in your body. First, exercise helps lower the levels of hormones such as cortisol and adrenaline. These are the hormones that trigger stress in the body or at least encourage it.

Further, it is pointed out that exercise helps encourage the production of endorphins. Endorphins are also commonly known as "feel good" chemicals of the body. This is because they are considered natural painkillers and mood elevators to the body. They are also responsible for promoting "runner's high" and the feelings of relaxation that you get every time you are done with a hard workout or a taxing physical activity.

The other explanation is that exercise helps you break out of your ordinary schedule. Working out provides you with an opportunity to "escape" and have the opportunity for recreation and free yourself from having to deal with the normal worries of life. This has the capacity of lowering your stress levels to some extent.

2. How working can help out with insecurity

Working out also helps with feelings of insecurity.

If you think about it, most of the time, insecurity stems from a deeply regarded belief and fear that you are being judged negatively in one way or another by those around you. And one reason you may have this belief or experience the fear may have to do with your physical appearance, or in other words, your self-image.

If you are like most people and haven't been living a healthy lifestyle, you probably worry that you are not physically appealing, are unfit, overweight or some variation of that. This can have a huge negative impact on your self-esteem and confidence, especially in public and social situations.

If that is the case, then working out could be the answer to your problems.

Picture yourself being totally different than you are right now physically. Imagine yourself with six pack abs, an athletic body, a flat tummy, great posture, balanced weight and anything else that society loves to obsess over.

Now imagine how that would make you feel deep down as compared to how you feel now. If the thought makes you feel better, then you can see how working out can help with your insecurities.

In addition, the sense of accomplishment will make you feel even better. How do you feel the moment you accomplish a certain project that took you a great deal of time and effort? The same goes for when you set a goal for your workout efforts and set out to achieve it. Doing so helps you feel better about yourself and this helps fight off your insecurities.

Conclusion

Whew! We have now come to the concluding part of this book.

Throughout this book, my objective has been to provide you with a fresh perspective on how working out can be approached. I have also pointed out the differences in what compels you to work out or achieve any goal in the first place. On top of that, I have also provided you with a variety of workout techniques to put into use.

It is my hope that this book has helped motivate you towards taking action in a better way that will help you accomplish your personal fitness goals and alleviate your stress insecurities.

What I encourage you to do from now on is to read this book over and over until you are certain that you've had a firm grasp of its true message. Afterwards, follow up what you read with action since that is the best way of getting the most out of this book.

Finally, I want to thank you for choosing to buy this book despite there being several out there on the same topic. Thanks once more and may you be blessed.

If you found the book valuable, can you recommend it to others? One way to do that is to post a review on Amazon.

Click here to leave a review for this book on Amazon!

Thank you and good luck!

www.ingramcontent.com/pod-product-compliance
Lightning Source LLC
Chambersburg PA
CBHW051426250726
48655CB00003B/1251